ESSAYS IN VACCINOLOGY

Prof.Dr.Ibrahim M S SHNAWA

Department of Biotechnology

College of Biotechnology

University of Qasim

Qasim ,Babylon

IRAQ.

PREFACE

Spending three decades of my scientific life in teaching immunology[20 years] and vaccinology[10 years] at University of Babylon and University of Qasim ,Babylon Governerate/IRAQ., for biology and biotechnology students. During the time I wrote ;Vaccine And Sera[Arabic] published by Dijla and Al Wedah publisher Aman/Jordan,2015,Vaccinology At A Glance, Lap Lambert,2016,Vaccinology Letters: A Treatise Concerning Experimental Vaccines, Create Space,2016,The Competing Experimental Bacterin Combinations ,Lap Lambert,2018.What remains in my edited deposit handout a series of reviews published in relevant scientific journals .I coined them in one monograph entitled "Essays In Vaccinology".The text handles the topics; Immunity To Vaccine, Animal Cell Based Vaccine ,And Vaccine Allied Biologics. Such monograph is intended to serve students and researchers in immunology , vaccinology and biotechnology fields.

Prof.Dr.Ibrahim Shnawa,Ph.D.
March,2018.

CONTENTS

I-Immunity To Vaccine	4-20
1-Overview	5-5
2-Cryglobulinemia Associated Immune Response To Vaccine.	6-10
3-Herd Immunity	11-20
II-Animal Cell Based Vaccine	21-35
4-Dendritic Cell Based Vaccine For Human Tuberculosis	22-35
III-Vaccine Allied Products	36-67
5-Vaccine Allied Biologics I	37-51
6-Vaccine Allied Biologics II	52-54
7-Immune Potentials Of Probiotics.	55-67

IMMUINITY TO VACCINE

> Vignette
> Vaccine stimulates an immune conversion state from baseline immunity to the clinically significant immune response in vaccinee during post-vaccination state. It induces; natural, immune cross road and adaptive humoral ,cellular ,humoral-cellular and/or autoimmunity as well as hypersensitivity responses. At rare instances ,however, it may pose to suppression ,anergy or tolerance state. Humoral immune responses may be in form of normo-globulin and/or cryoglobulin.

IMMUNITY TO VACCINE: AN OVERVIEW

1-Concept : It is a preparation derived from human or animal pathogen(s), may be the virulence determinants ,make it available for prevention or therapy of infectious diseases of man and animals.

2-Preparation: Vaccine can be prepared from :live microbe, attenuated pathogens ,microbial subunits or that manufactured via molecular techniques.

3-Types: They are of several types such as heat killed ,live ,live attenuated ,subunits ,conjugate as well as molecular vaccines.

4-Immunological basis of vaccine action :Active host immune system, active primed memory B and T cells ,establishment of immune-conversion

5-Evaluation: There are several criteria that are helpful in the evaluation of the prepared vaccine, the most important of which are: Purity homogeneity ,shelf life, toxicity ,antigenicity, immunogenicity ,and immune effectivity.

6-Failiure: Vaccine fail either by the cause of the host immune system defects or the host is *genetically in susceptible to the vaccine. Meanwhile ,the failure of the vaccine may be due to its nature per see in which non-homogeniety ,expiry, toxicity and impurities.*

7-Side effects :*Several side effects are familiar to be occurred following vaccination program like ;fever ,hypersensitivity. secondary cryoglobulinemia and/or an autoimmune responses.*

BACTERIN INDUCED PATHOGENIC LAPIN AND MURINE CRYOGLOBULINS

ABSTRACT

The nature of the mammalian humoral immunoglobulin responses to antigens in general are either one or more than one of the followings; mono-partite[nomoglobulin],dipartite [normoglobulin ,cryoglobulin] and /or tripartite [normoglobulin ,cryoglobulin ,pyroglobulin] .While,for bacterin it can be monopartite [normoglobulin] ,dipartite [normogloblin ,cryglobulin].Three experimental settings have been adopted. Bacterin induced cryoglobulin responses in turn may induce cryoglobulin specific pathogenic potentials as that noted in cases of BCG[pneumogenic, nephritogenic ,lymphogenic and granulomatogenic] and Salmonella typhi [pneumogenic ,nephritogenic ,lymphogenic] bacterin induced cryoglobulin in lapin and murine laboratory animal models .Such pathology is standing as interfering side effect in the preclinical experimental vaccine evaluation studies. Bacterin during vaccination programs might be of potential cause for cryoglobulin induced pathogenicity in vaccinee.

Key Words: Antigen ,Bacterin, cryoglobulin,interference,Preclinical.

INTRODUCTION

The systemic humoral mammalian immune responses to antigens[Table,1] span between normoglobulin,cryoglobulin and / or pyroglobulin(1,2).While for bacterins it can be normoglobulin and / or cryglobulin(3,4).The objective of the present opinion was to affix cryoglobulin induced pathology as a consequences of bacterin immunization.

EXPERIMENTAL SETTINGS
Three experimental settings have been adopted;
Setting I: BCG induced(5),S.typhi induced(6)and B.melitensis induced (3) in a lapin animal models.
Setting II :S.typhi induced cryglobulin mediated pathology (7) in a lapin models.
Setting III: Human tuberculus cryoglobulin induced pathology in murine model (8).

IMMUNOFIXATION
The immunofixation studies have shown mixed cryoglobulinemia of IgM-IgG-IgA in typhoid vaccinee and typhoid patients(9) and mixed two variant cryoglobulin responses were noted among Brucella patients as IgM-IgG-IgA and IgM-IgG[Table,2] responses(10).

PATHOGENICITY
It has been found that human and lapin S typhi cryglobulin was pneumogenic ,nephritogenic , and lyphogenic in rabbits model (7).While. human tuberuclus tuberculus cryoglobulin was pneumogenic ,nephritogenic,lymphogenic and granulomatogenic[Table,3] in murine model (8).

BOOSTING
The adopted bacterin priming for rabbit and mice depends on a starting dose then two successive boosting dose at a week a part. It has been found that the more exposure to bacterin the more cryoglobulin producing and the more cryglobulin pathogenicity(7,8).

MECHANISM
Bacterin specific immune-priming induced normoglobulin and cryoglobulin responses. Cryoglobulin in turn induced specific pathogenicity (7,8).

INTERFERENCE

Bacterin induced pathogenicity may interferes with safety[Table,4] parameter of vaccine candidate preclinical evaluation parameters in laboratory animal level.

CONCLUSIONS

Bacterins on specific immune priming of lapin and murine animal models produce ,normoglobulin and cryoglobulin responses. Allogenic and xenogenic cryoglobulin has been found to be pneumogenic ,nephritogenic and lymphogenic.A point to be noted when any candidate bacterin is going to be evaluated in laboratory animal models for approval to human health welfare .

Table 1 :Systemic Humoral immune responses to antigens and bacterins [1,2]

Response type	Response Nature for antigen	Response nature for bacterin
Monopartite	Normoglobulin	Normoglobulin
Dipartite	Normoglobulin ,Cryoglobulin	Normoglobulin ,Cryoglobulin
Tripartite	Normoglobulin ,Cryglobulin ,Pyrogglobulin	

Table 2 : Cryoglobulin Isotypes in human Patients.

Human Disease Type	Cryoglobulin Nature	References
Typhoid Vaccinee ,Typhoid Patients	IgM-IgG-IgA	(9)
Brucella Pre-immune ,Brucella Patients	IgM-IgG-IgA ,IgM-IgG	(10)

Table 3 : Cryoglobulin Pathogenicity(11).

Animal Model	Cryoglobulin Source	Pathogenicity
Lapin	Human,Lapin	Pneumogenic, Nephritogenic, Lymphogenic (7)
Murine	Human	Pneumogenic, Nephritogenic,Lymphogenic, Granulomatogenic(8)

Table 4 : Preclinical Evaluation of Bacterins and limits of Cryoglobulin interference(12).

Evaluation Parameters	Interference
I-Cell culture Studies Safety Antigenicity	- -
Laboratory Animal Studies Safety Antigenicity Immunogenicity Immune Protectivity	+ - - -

+ = Interference

References
1-Parslow TG , Stites DP , Terr AI , Imboden JB,2001.Medical Immunology 10th ed.Lange Medical books/McGraw –Hill NY,218-219.
2-Shnawa IMS,2014,Pyroglobulinemia and human Arthropathy,WJPR,3(7):45-48.
3-Shnawa IMS , Jassim Y A,2016,Lapin cryoglobulin responses to Brucella meletensis RV-1,IJAPB 5(3):341-345.
4-Shnawa IMS,2016,Vaccinology Letters : A Treatise Concerning Experimental Vaccines ,IISTE ,USA .
5-Shnawa IMS , Jassim Y A ,2011,BCG and tuberculin induced experimental secondary cryogobuinemia ,OMJ,7(12):209-219.
6-Shnawa IMS ,ALSerhan A J ,2014,The Immune features of S typhi somatic O antigen induced lapin cryoglobulinemia, Int.J.Curr.Res.,6(10):9065-9068.
7-Shnawa IMS ,ALSerhanAJ,2014,The Pathogenic Potentials of S typhi specific human and lapin cryoglobulin in a lapin model, Int.res.J.Biol.Sci.,3(5):57-61.
8-ALZamily KY,Shnawa IMS,ALAzawi A J-R,2017,An immune mediated and tissue responses induced by human tuberculus cryoglobulin in murine model.,Kerb.J.Agri.Sci.(Special issue),accepted.
9-Shnawa IMS ,ALSerhan AJ,2014,Mixed IgG,IgM,IgA cryoglobulin responses in human typhoid patients IOSR,JPBS,9(2):26-29.
10- Shnawa IMS,Jassim Y A ,2014,Mixed two variant types of cryoglobulinemia associated with brucellosis human patients,WJPR,3(4):1883-1889.
11-Shnawa IMS,2015,Immunology of Natural And Induced Cryoglobulinemia,IISTE,USA.
12-National Institute of Health,1998,Understanding Vaccines Publication Number 98-4219.

Human herd Immunity

Abstract

Herd is facing insults[stimulants], like; concurrent, present, past or forthcoming infections and/or vaccinations. Such insults are the inducers for the immune conversion from naïve B or naïve T or both into effector or memory lymphocytes. The herd immune response to these insults can be as; high, moderate low and/or non. Herd immunity plots CD4+ and CD8+ lymphocytes counts, IL12 P40, as well as S.typhi H specific antibody titers were given as study cases where human herd immunity do operate in which both Gaussian distribution curve and skewing plots were evident.

Key Words; Herd ,Herd Immunity ,infection

Introduction

Individual forming the population[herd] and environment interplayed mutual influential effects on each other(John&Smuel 2000).The individual is single autonomus biological system that performs various biotic activities which render it viable within its own population or herd. It is either uni, or multicellular organism(Hallgrimssion & Brain 2011) The letteral meaning of variation is the difference occurred between one another within same molecule, organelle, organism. Such variation can be of adaptive or genetic type(Crawford et al.2007).

Variations within the individuals; These variations are mainly of molecular and cellular nature .Leukocyte antigen genes, erythrocyte antigen genes as well as immunoglobulin gene families, immunoglobulin allotypes and ideotypes .The genetic variations are including gene copy number variation, single nucleotide polymorphism. These molecular variations are either of genes or proteins in nature and are forming the major determinants of human herd immunity .Cellular variations can be of common occurrence in lymphocytes such as B1,B2,B10,Th1,Th2,Th9,Th22.(Tan,Gery.2012,Tesmer et al2008,Eyerich et al2009,Palomares et al 2010) As well as;A1,A2,B,BH,AB,H(Bryant1982,Tizzard 2012,Lewis et al. 2001). Variations among individuals: Human individuals forming a herd do variate in one or more of the followings; HLA type, Erythrocyte type ,Allotype as well as ideotype. Such single or combined variations may be of influencial effects on disease susceptibility(Boyed et al3). Herd constitute a number of individuals forming a population harboring certain geographic place affecting on another and affecting their environment .The environment ,however, may in turn affect them. Such interacting biotic and abiotic factors forms a community together with the place they will form the niche. A niche can be ,hospital ward ,military camp or a school class room(Jone&Smuel 2000).Herd Immunity is of three relevant fraction or fractions of the individuals forming the herd who are immune against certain infectious disease .Such immunities are resulting from ;pre immunity ,vaccination or infection(Ali et al.,2005,John& Smuel 2000,Fine 1993).

What determine the herd immunity is the dominance nature of MHS ,Ig gene sets, erythrocyte antigen genes, limits of parasitism, past vaccination program as well as the limits of cellular immune conversion of the main ,B or T lymphocytes into effectors and/or memory phenotypes These all together determine the baseline natural and adaptive immune functions(John &Smuel 2000;Newman&Antczack 1983).The degree of responses of the individuals within a human herd can be in one of four classes ;High responder ,moderate responder ,low responder and non-responder .These classes are generally encoded by the MHS system(Newman&Antczack1983).

Herd Immunity Plots

The mathematical modulation of human herd immunity are mostly represented by the Guassian distribution curves ;At times ,however, skewing do happened in such distributon(Steel et al .1998).

1-CD4+vsCD8+ lymphocytes; The numbers of CD4+T cells were used to plot the herd immunity curve. It was with an apparent skewing patterns.TheCD8+T cell count were showing normal distribution curve Figures 1,2(Shnawa, et al. 2009).

2-Cytokine:IL12 P40 was detected in 18 pulmonary tuberculosis patients and plotted.The plot was with an evident skewing patternFigure3(Shnawa et al.,2013).

3-Salmonella typhi antiH :S.typhi anti-H titres were used to map herd immunity curve among enteric fever patients .The plot looks like normal distribution curve(Shnawa &Hindi 1996,Lloyd-Smith et al.,2005).

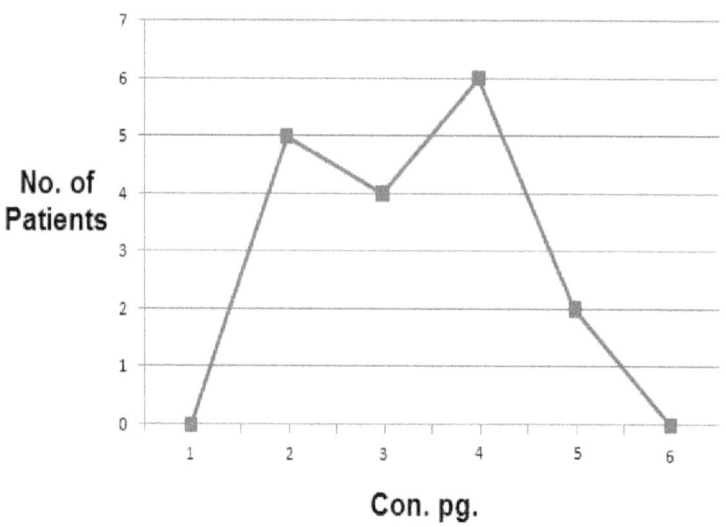

Figure 1
IL12 P40 as a probe for herd immunity

IL12 P40 in PTB
1 – 0   0
2 – 1-200   5
3 – 201-400   4
4 – 401-600   6
5 – 601-800   3
6 – 801-1000   0

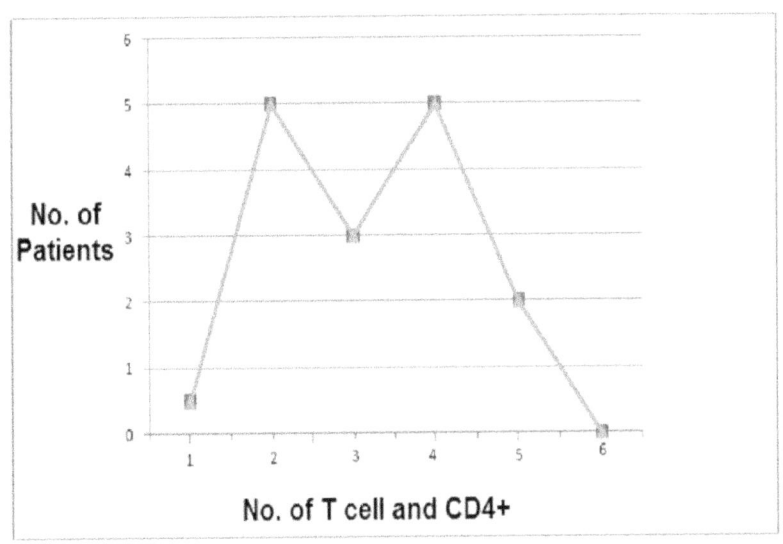

Figure 2 : CD4+ as a probe for herd immunity

1 – 300-599   0
2 – 600-899   5
3 – 900-1200   3
4 – 901-1500   5
5 – 1501-1800   2
6 – 1801-2001   0

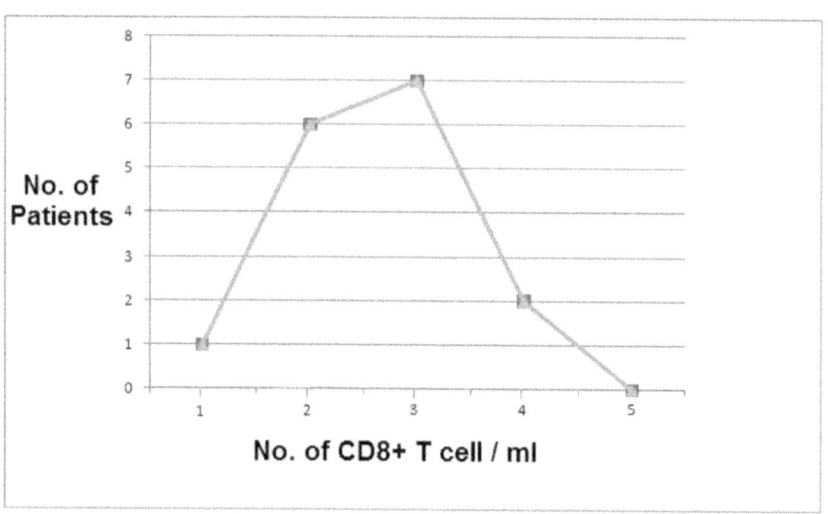

Figure 3: CD8 as a probe for human herd immunity

1 – 1-300   0
2 – 301-600   6
3 – 601-900   7
4 – 901-1200   2
5 – 1201-1500   0

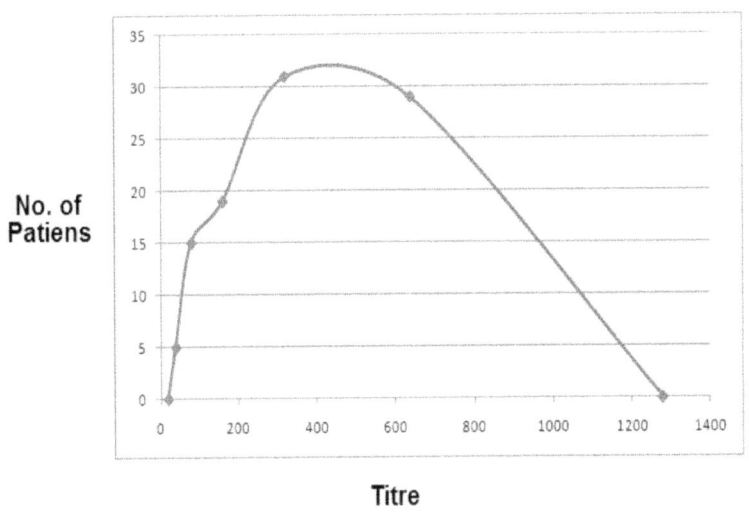

Figure 4:S.typhi anti-H as a probe of human herd

1 – 20   0
2 – 40   5
3 – 80   15
4 – 160   19
5 – 320   31
6 – 640   29
7 – 1280   0

Conclusion

CD4 ,CD8,IL12 P40 and S.typhi anti H antibody titres are helpful as a cprobe for infectious and tumor invasion in human herd and be useful in mapping herd immunity.Individuals foming the herd were of low,moderate and high response.The herd plots were either normal distribution or skewed type.

Acknowledgment

The author wish to express his gratitude to Prof .Hindi ,W,Ph.D .Techniqal institute, Babylon for his help when he had been the coordinator of Babylon board.

References
1-Ali M ,Emch M, Seidlein LV,Yunus M,Sack DA,Rao M,Homgren J,Clemen JD(2005).Herd immunity conferred by killed oral cholera vaccines in Bangladesh;reanalysis.Lancet366(9479):44-49.
2-Bryant NL(1982)An Introduction to Immunohaematology 2nd ed. WB Sounders Company ,Philadelphia.
3-BoyedSD,GaetaBA,Jackson KJ ,Fire AZ ,Marshall EL,others(2010).Individual variations in germline Ig gene rearrangement.Journal ofImmunology.184,6986-6992.
4-Brisson M,Van de Velde ,FrancoELF ,DoletM ,Bioly M-C (2011)Incremental impact of adding boys to current human Papillomavirus vaccination programs ;Role of herd immunity.Journal ofInfectousDisease.204(3),372-376.

5-Crawford DL, Oleksiak MF(2007)The biological importance of measuring individual variations.Journal of Experimental Biology.210(Pt.9),1613-1621
6=EyerichS ,Eyerich K, Pennino D, &others(2009).Cells represent a distinct human T cell subset involved in epidermal immunity and remodeling .Journal of.Clinical.Investigation.119(12),2573-2585.
7-Fine PEM (1993).Herd Immunity;History,Theory,practice.Epidemiol.Rev.15(2):265-302.
8-Hallgrimsson ,Brain K(2011).Variation ,A cenral concept in Biology.Academic Press,Science.
9-John TJ, Smuel R (2000).Herd immunity and Herd effect;New insight and definition.Eur.J.Epidemiol.16(7):601-606.
10-Lloyd-Smith JO, Schreiber SJ, Kopp& PE,Getz WM (2005):Superspreading and effect of individual variations on disease.Nature 438:355-359.
11-Lewis SM,Bain BJ,&BatesI(2001).Dacie and Lewis s Practical Haematology,9thed Chuchill-Livingstone ,London.
12-Newman MJ&,Antczack DF(1983). Histocompatability polymorphism ofDomestic animals.Advances in Veterinary $cience and Comparative Medcine.27,1-76.
13-Palomares,O,Yaman G,Azkar AK ,Akkoc T,Europian Journal ofImmunology 40,1232-1240.
14-Roitte I,Brostoff J&,Male D(2001).Immunology 6th ed.Mosby,London,435.
15-Steel RGD, Torrie JH &,Dickey DA (1997).Principles And Procedures of statistics:A biometrical Approach,3rd ed. McGraw Hill Series in probability and Statistics,NewYork,1-8.
16-Shnawa IMS& ,Hindi WAZ(1996).febrile circulating agglutinins .The Technologist 31:29-36.

17-Shnawa IMS ,ALMaliky KA,& AlMersomy HD(2009).CD4/CD8 ratio, CEA and Ca 15-3 as abattery for diagnosis of women breast cancer. Medical Journal of Babylon.6(2),339-349.

18-Shnawa IMS, AlMamuri RTO ,&Mohammed G.J.(2013).The assessment of IL12P40 among primary pulmonary and chronic(old) tuberculosis.International Research Journal of Biological Science.2(12),1-4.

19-Tan C & Gery L.(2012)Unique features of Th9 cells and their products.Critical Review of Immunology 32,1-10.

20-Tesmer LA,Lundy SK,Sarkar& S,Fox DA (2008).Th17 cells in human diseases.ImmunologyReview223,87-113.

21-Tizzard I(2012).An Introduction To Veterinary Immunology.9th ed.WBSaunders.

ANIMAL CELL BASED VACCINE

> **Vignette**
>
> Mammalian cell can be of use in vaccine production. The gene or genes encoding specific protein(s) containing the bacterial virulence determinant can be isolated and transfected to mammalian cell in culture. Then the transfected cells can be exploited to produce large quantities of the protein which can be developed into highly purified subunit vaccine. Two trends may be usable as:
>
> i-Ex-vivo involves the isolation of the subject leukocytes, culturing them in suitable cell culture system. Then the gene encodes for specific immune-dominant virulence epitope is transfected to these cells and reintroduced to the subject.
>
> ii-In-vivo approach in which direct injection of the gene encoding the immune-dominant virulence epitope into resident tissue or organs through retro or adeno-associated vector to facilitate insertion of the gene.

DENDRITIC CELL BASED VACCINE FOR HUMAN TUBERCULOSIS :

ABSTRACT

Immune cells may serve for vaccine technology and for gene therapy. They are basically of lymphocyte and dendritic cell types. These cells can be of adoptive and educated forms .Dendritic cell based vaccine technology can be established through ;In-vitro, ex-vivo and/or in-vivo procedures. Subunit target antigen loading onto DCs or through insertion of gene construct cloned into a specific viral or plasmid vectors .Dendritic cell based vaccine designs are found of use for infectious and cancer diseases .Experimental dendritic cell based vaccine specific for ;viral ,bacterial ,fungal and protozoal infectious diseases are being ongoing in current research. Tuberculosis in man and animals is problematic at worldwide scale including our country. The approved BCG vaccine is being of questionable efficacy in infants, immune-compromised and pulmonary tuberculosis patients .The SO2 attenuated live tuberculosis vaccine is in its way for clinical trials .Experimental dendritic cell based vaccine designs specific for tuberculosis are being of educated DCs loaded with the target protein ,peptide or trans-fected with gene construct codes for these proteins .Laboratory animal immune evaluations have found to be the inserted gene DC is superior to antigen loaded Dc based vaccines in sense of immune protectivity. The current layout of tuberculosis vaccine is; BCG questioned ,SO2 is being in its way for clinical trials and DC-based vaccine still experimental. Approved Dc based tuberculosis preventive and therapeutic forms are still the near future goal of vaccinologists all over the world.

Key Words: Adopted, Dendritic cell, educated, Ex-vivo ,in-vivo, technology, Vaccine.

1-Introduction;
Dendritic cell serves critical vaccine adjuvant or vaccine design for prevention and /or treatment of microbial infections ,allograft rejection treatment of cancer and autoimmune diseases[1].The objective of the present mini-review is to sum-up the current attitude about the Dc based vaccine for tuberculosis, the rather common disease in this area and all over the world knowing that In 2015.10.4million people became ill with tuberculosis around the world , and 1.8 million related death ,95% of which occur in the low and middle income countries [2,3,4,5,6] .

2-Phylogeny:
As a phagocyte and phagocytosis in turn, they definitely appeared as functional professional phagocytes in earth worm with coelum passing through the evolutionary animal group ranks up to vertebrate[7] .Boney fish devoted from bone marrow with an evident extra-medullary heamopoiesis[8] .From amphibian up to mammals, bone marrow haemopoiesis were evident[6].In boney fish ,however. mononuclear cell system appeared as Melano-macrophage centres in spleen and in liver [9,10,11] .

3-Ontogeny:
Tracing the ontogeny of the mononuclear cell system ,it is rooted back to embryonic yolk sac, then fetal liver and fetal bone marrow during the embryonic life of the fetus. They arose as pluri-potent stem cells [12,13] .

4-Stem Cells:

The embryonic stem cells are; self re-newable ,multi-potent ,and non-differentiate cells with a set of characteristic surface markers .These surface markers can be changed on differentiation to definite cell entity. Such cells have the ability to be differentiated to any cell type in accordance with the surrounding micro-environmental tissue mellue .Among these cell entities are the mononuclear cell system [14].

5-Macrophages:

Macrophage is a general term denoted to all cells of the mononuclear cell system that have phagocytic activity. Mononuclear cell system(MCS) is a group of human and mammalian leukocytes harboring peripheral blood and the reticculo-endothelial organs ,with rather different surface markers, Table 1.They performed an array of immunobiologic functions[6]. Mature mononuclear cell forms and functions varies in accordance with their own surrounding tissue microenvironment Their nomenclature will be; glail, alveolar ,kupffer ,dendritic ,Langerhans, monocyte and osteoclasts harboring ;brain, lung ,liver, lymph node and bone marrow ,skin, blood and bone respectively [15,16,17].The MCS displayed the functions of; uptake, process, present and immune recognize the antigens as a preliminary step in the immune response events .

In ,Pyres patchs ,MCS have the antigen delivered by M cells, they take up and present it to helper T cells then triggering B or T cell responses. At the lymph node interdigitating dendritic cell delivered antigens directly presenting them to B lymphocytes to initiate immune response events. Langerhans cells are skin defenders .Kupffer cells in liver on antigenic stimulation undergoes shape changes and increase in numbers within the liver paranchyma and contribute to the local liver immunity against the invading pathogens[18] .Resting alveolar macrophage in lung tissue melliue are small ovoid in active, on stimulation they appeared larger in size and becomes rather ameboid in shape[18] .Glail cells in brain and CNS tissues during infectious invasion undergoes cell form changes to satellite appearance, increase in numbers and produce cytokines as well as contribute in tissue regeneration[19] .

Osteoclast contribute in bone tissue catabolism. Monocytes are phagocytic ,antigen presenting, cytokine producer and might be differentiated into immature dendritic cells then to mature dendritic by local cytokine action[13].MCS, form the model systems for testing; phagocytosis, macrophage inhibitory factor, ex-vivo cytokine production and antibody production by B lymphocyte[20,21,22].

6-Dendritic Cells:
DC is satellite in shape with irregular nucleus in mature form and bean shaped nucleus and ameboid shaped in the immature form. DCs are professional phagocytes and acting as antigen presenting cells(APC).They process antigens through MHCI,MHCII and CD1 pathways .

DCs circulating within the host capture and deliver microbial and/or cancer cell subunit antigens. Their circulation starts from lymphoid tissue to peripheral blood and back to lymphoid tissue. DCs differentiation path starts with lympho-myeloid progenitor cells to pro-monocyte immature monocyte then to mature monocyte .From monocyte by the effect of cytokine to immature DCs then to mature DCs. The surface marker for both mature and immature is basically the same but with marked quantitative differences, Table 2 ,DCs are hetero-genus group of cells that displayed difference in various anatomic sites ,cell surface phenotypes and functions. Thus ,its sub-grouped into three subsets, Table 3 .DCs expressed a sort of cell plasticity[23,24,25].

7-Dendritic Cell Technology:

Immune cells can be of use for vaccine or gene therapy technologies. The most tempted immune cell types were lymphocytes and dendritic cells[26,27,28].These cells are either in adopted or educated forms. Hence several technologic trends are currently useable for educating DCs to be valid as a base for vaccine technology both for preventive and therapeutic vaccine types .Details of the DCs based vaccine technology are being stated in the followings;

i-Blood samples with anti-coagulants collected from patients .dendritic cells are separated, purified and incubated with the subunit antigen of the causal and re-injected back to the patients[29].

ii-Ex-vivo approach involves the separation purification and culturing of DCs in cell culture system. Then the target gene construct is added through an appropriate vector to facilitate its journey to the appropriate target cells[29].

iii- Blood samples with an anti-coagulant collected from the patients, dendritic cells are separated, purified and cultured in cell culture system in presence of antigen source, loading agent ,maturation agent[23] .

iv-In-vivo within the host, antigen targeted to dendritic cell through binding to ICAM3 DCs sign or to CD209 establishing promising in-vivo loading of antigens to DCs[30].

8-Dendritic Cell Based Vaccines :

For an effective DC-based vaccine designs development against polio, measles, and hepatitis B. These vaccines composed of microbial antigens are often made with adjuvant ,Table 4 , that activate DCs .There are urgent need for both preventive and therapeutic vaccine for tuberculosis replacing the currently blamed as ineffective the BCG [31].Since till now no approved dendritic cell based tuberculosis vaccine are developed, evaluated and licensed. However several experimental Dc based tuberculosis vaccine tested iv-vitro, ex-vivo and in-vivo to the rank of laboratory animal evaluations are being documented all over the world[23,30,31,32].

9-DCs based vaccine induced Immune Conversion;

The M tuberculosis is obliged intracellular pathogen on invasion of the host it will stimulate Th1 or Th1 and TH2 responses[33] at the week 4 up to the week 12,the immune conversion sought as cytokine rise in concentration and/or specific antibody concentration or titres together with immune protection percentages .Here we abstracting two experimental vaccination protocols in laboratory animal models to give a clue to the nature of post vaccination immune conversions.

i-Three groups of mice were the test laboratory animals;first wa vaccinated with DC loaded with Ag85,the second with DC loaded CD4/Cd8 T cell peptide and the third vaccinated with adeno-virus cloned with Ag85 gene transfected to DCs. The group of IL12 and was more immunogenic than group one and two. Comparing the first group to the second and third. The third elicited a remarkably higher levels of ex-vivo INFg at the weeks 2,6 and 12 post-immunization which was paralleled with high frequency of Antigen specific T cells[34].

ii- Two groups of mice were the test laboratory animal.The first immunized with calf Mtbag-calf serum –Dcs vaccine and the second immunized with Mtb ag-mouse serum-DCs vaccine in a three doses protocol, animal was watched in first ,second and third dose in both groups for bacillary load after challenge, INFg level, survival and immune protection percentages. The second group have shown reduced bacillary load in lungs and spleen, increase of survival times, and as well as increase of INfg producing cells in lung and lymphoid tissue .DC based vaccine group two pays critical role in induction of protective immunity against M tuberculosis challenge[35].

10-Dendritic cell based vaccine Evaluations ;
NHI in here monograph published in 1998 [36],"Understanding Vaccines" have been put-forward set of criteria for evaluation of prototype or candidate vaccines in this paragraph we apply this set of criteria onto tuberculosis DC based vaccine and the evaluation layout is depicted in the table 5 .

Table 1 : The Cell Surface Markers of the Macrophages[6,37]

Cell marker	Langerhans cell	Interdittating Cell	Follicular DCs	GCDC	Macrophagic
MHCII	+	+	-	+	+/-
CD32	+	-	+	+	+
CD64	+/-	-	-	-	+
CR1	+	-	+	+	+
CD21	-	-	high	Low	+
CD1a	+	-	-	-	-
CD40	?	High	+	Low	+

DC = Dendritic cells   GCDC= Germinal Centre Dendritic Cells.

Table 2: Cell surface and intracellular markers of mature and immature DCs.[24]

DC stage/ Surface markers	MHCII Molecule	CD54, CD58, CD88, CD86	CD40CD25 IL12	CD83, P55	Granule antigen	M3242A1 MIO38
Immature	High Intracell	Low	Low	Low	Low	Normal
Mature	High Surface	High	High	High	High	Low

Table 3 : Dendritic Cell subset characteristics[24]

pDCs subset	One	CD303,CD1C,CD14, C type lectin,Surface and intracellular TLR,Intracellular Helicases
mDC subset	Two	Reciprocal CD1C,CD14,MHCI,XCL1 C type lectin,Surface and intacellular TLR,Intrcellular helicases

Table 4:DCs based vaccines for infectious diseases[1,31,38]

Microbial Agent	DC based construct Inserted Vaccine	DC based antigen loaded Vaccine
Virus	HIV,LCMV,EHV-1	Poliovirus, Measlesvirus,HepatitisB virus
Bacteria	Chlamydia Sp. M,tuberculosis Borrelia burgdorferi	M.tuberculosis P.aruginosa
Protozoa	Toxoplasma gondi L.donovani	
Fungi ,Oppotunistic	Candida sp.[38]	

Table 5: Evaluation of DCbased Vaccine for human tuberculosis

NIH criteria 1998[29]	BCG vaccine[40]	SO2 vaccine[39]	DCs gene Construct vaccine[34]	DC antigen loaded Vaccine[34]
Understanding Disease	+	+	+	+
Understanding Disease agent	+	+	+	+
Developing Vaccine candidate: Safety Identity Antigenicity Immunogenicity	+ + + +	+ + + +	+ + ++ ++	+ + + +
Testing Vaccine in Volunteers Phase I Phase II Phase III	+ + +	To be tested	Still	Still

11-Dendritic Cell Based Vaccine In Brief:

The developed and laboratory animal evaluated experimental DC based vaccine for tuberculosis own several immune features depicted in the following points

i-Gene construct inserted DC based tuberculosis vaccine are more immunogenic and more protective than antigen loaded DC vaccines.

ii-Mouse serum is better adjuvant than calf serum Dc based tuberculosis vaccine in mouse model for immune conversion parameters.

iii-The laboratory animal evaluation parameters include INFg, IL12,reduction in bacillary load, survival time, and immune protection percent.

iv-Subcutaneous rout is rather better than ,intramuscular ,and intravenous routs for DC based vaccine for tuberculosis.

v-The general vaccine NIH 1998 evaluation parameters are being partly applicable on DC based vaccine for tuberculosis.

vi-The current tuberculosis vaccine layout is being as; BCG questioned,SO2 in its way for clinical evaluation and DC-based vaccine is still experimental.

References:

1-Lipscomb F,Masten BJ,2002,Dendritic cells:Immune Regulators in health and disease,Physiol.Rev.:82:97-130.
2-Shnawa,IMS,ALMukhtar S,Adoos SA,2005,Mass surveillance of pediatric tuberculosis exposure using dermal tuberculin reactivity as a tracer,Kufa Med.J.8(1):104-110.
3-AlSaadi,MAK,Shnawa IMS,ALMukhtar S,2007,An evaluation study of cellular immunological functions in anergic tuberculus patients.Med.J.Baby.4(3-4):198-204.
4-Sawa MI, Shnawa IMS ,ALHassan AJ ,Circulating Immunoglobulin levels in patints with pulmonary tubeculusis,Iraq.Med.J.36(1):32-380
5-WHO,2016,Tuberculosis Fact Sheet ,Media Centre.
6-Owen JA, Punt J, Stranford SA,2013Kuby Immunology,7th ed,,Macmillian ,Higher Education ,New York,27-40.
7-Playfair JHL, Chain BM,2001,Immunology,At A Glance,7th ed.,Blackwell Science. com,Tehran,12-13.

8-Roberts RD,2012,Fish Pathology,4th ed.,Wiley Black.
9-Pronina SV, Batueva MDD ,Pronina NM,2014, Chracateristics of melanomacrophage centres in the spleen and liver of the Rutilus rutilu (Cypriforms,Cypridae) in the lack Kotokel during the Haff disease outbreaks,J.Ecthilogy,54(1):104-110.
10-=Aqius C, Roberts RJ ,2003,Melanomarphage centres and their role in fish pathology,J.Fish dis. ,26 (9):499-509.
11-ALNiaeem KS,Shnawa IMS,ALSadi B A E,2015,The immunological responses for spleen as a biomarker against Aeromonas hydrophila in Cyprinus carpio,Bas. Vet. Med.J.,15(2):306-315.
12-Hume DA,2006,The mononuclear Phagocyte System. Curr .Opin.
Immunol .,18(1):49-53.
13-Hume,2008,Differentiation and heterogeneity in the mononuclear phagocyte system,Mucosal .Immunol.1(6):432-441.
14-Tuch BE,Stem cells – a clinical update,Aust Fam.Physician,35(9):719-721.
15-Davis P,1984,The mononuclear Phagocytes,In,Dale MM,Foreman JC,textbook Of Immunopharmacology,Blackwell Scientific Publication,Oxford,79-92.
16-Gordon S,2006,Mononuclear Phagocyte,In Male D , Brostoff I , Roth DB, Roitt I, 7th ed.Mosby,Canada,181-202.
17-Shnawa IMS,Hassen AJ ,2002,An Age related enhancement of E.coli Reticulo-endothelial system clearance in a lapin model,Bay.Uni.J.,7(3):1008-1011.
18-Shnawa IMS ,ALZamily KY ,Omran R ,Alwan MJ,2014,Lympoid and lympho-myeloid hyperplasia and immune protection, JAPBC,3(4):901-911.
19-Shnawa,IMS,2014,The Identification of Anuran glial cell.,Int.Sci.Ind.,8(8):778-780.

20-Paulnock DM,2000,Macrphage,Practical Approach ,Oxford.
21-Stevens CD,2010,Clinical Immunology And Serology :A Laboratory Perspective,3rd ed.,FA Davis Company, Philadelphia.8-11.
22-Rose NR,Bigazzi PE ,1980,Methods In Immunodiagnosis,2nd ,ed.,Wiley Publication,USA,45-64.
23-Pizzarro GA,Barrio MM,2015,dendritic Cell based vaccine efficacy:aiming for hot spots,Front.Immunol.,6:1-8.
24-Palucko K , Banchereau J,2012,Cancer Immunotherapy,Nat.Rev.Can.,12,265-277.
25-Banchereau J,Steinman RM,1998,Dendritic cell and control of immunity, Nature:245-252.
26-Kong X, Hu Y, Cai Z,Yang F, Zhang Q , 2015 , dendritic cell-based technology landscape;Insight from patents and citation network ,Human vaccines and Immunotherapy.,11(5):682-688.
27-Cintolo J,Data J,Czerniecki B ,2012,Dendritic cell based vaccines:barriers and opportunities,Fut.Oncol.,5:1273-1279.
28-Tabarkiewicz J,2012,Dendritic cell:Active and passive p[layers in therapy of human disease:Immunotherapy,4:975-978.
29-Adkinson LR,Brown D,2007,Elseviers Integrated Genetics,Mosby ,Philadelphia ,223.
30-Xiao L,2013,Dendritic Cell Specific Vaccine,utility of antibody-mini-legend and lentivirus System,Ph.D. Dessert,university of Southren Califorina.
31-Paluckara K, Banchereau J, Mellman I,2010,Desiging vaccines:Based on biology of human dendritic cell subsets,Immunity,33(4):464-478.
32-Nair SK,Tomaras GD,Sales AP et al.,2014, High throughput identification and dendritic cell based functional validation of MHCI restricted Mycobacterium tuberculosis epitopes,Scientific Reports 4,Article Number 4632.

33-Sinha A ,Salam N, Gupta S, Natarajan K,2007,Mycobacterium tuberculosis and Dendritic cells,recognition,activation and functional implications. ,Ind. J .Biochem .Biophysics.,44:279-288.
34-Malowany JI, McCormick S, Santouosso M et al.,2006,development of cell based tuberculosis vaccines: genetically modified dendritic cell much more potent activator of CD4 and CD8 T cells than peptide or protein loaded counterpart .Mol. Thera.,13(4):766.
35-Rubakova E et al.2007,Specificity and efficacy of dendritic cell based vaccination against Mycobacterium tuberculosis antigens in a mouse model,Tuberculosis,81(2):134-144.
36-NIH,1998,Understanding Vaccines ,Publication Number-98-4219,23.
37-Shnawa IMS,2014,Immunology,IShtar Publishing House,Jordan,98
38-Kundu G ,Noverr MC,2011,Exposure to host or fungal PGE2,abrogates protection following immunization with Candida-plused dendritic cells, Med. Mycol.,49:380-394.
39-Enta et al.,2014,A Human dendritic cell based in-vitro model to assess Mycobaterium tuberculosis SO2 vaccine immunogenicity ,ALKTEX,31(4/14):397-406.
40-Shnawa IMS,2016,Vaccinology At A Glance,Lab lambert Acaedmic Press, Germany.

VACCINE ALLIED PRODUCTS

> Vignette
>
> Vaccine allied products are standard biologics that have vaccine immune features but they are of different nature than the classical known vaccine types. The may include;
>   i-Cancer killing Bacteria
>   ii-Genetically modified cancer killing bacteria
>   iii-Cancer killing T lymphocytes
>   iv-Probiotics.

VACCINE ALLIED BIOLOGICS-I

Abstract

Since the down of human civilization that might begin with Chinese and Indian tradition in curing human as well as animal diseases they had had been using variety of remedies (Therapeutics) originated from both animal and plant resources. The human need for therapeutics led him almost always searching for new preparations . Now it is being an opportunity to gather hetero-genus preparations in a group-wise fashion as that of vaccine like, standard or standardized immune-biologics which have some features of vaccines in one proposed group designated as therapeutic vaccine allied biologics(TVAB) .To date it is being evident the proposal holding that at least there are five classes of(TVAB) available both at experimental level and to a lesser extent to the level of clinical use .The classes are as; cellular secretions(cytokines ,antibodies) ,receptor-anti-receptor(immune check point inhibitors) , subunit macromolecules (Beta Glucan) and commensal microbiome(probiotics) and Bacterio-therapeutics(cancer killing bacteria) . These proposed classes were evaluated by vaccine criteria as well as by a group specific special evaluation criteria ,collectively ,it is being a state of developing a novel evaluation system. They are helpful as therapeutics for ;microbial ,envenomation ,immune mediated and neoplastic diseases with variable degrees of success .

Key Words: Antibody, Bacterio-therpeutics, Biologics ,cellular , cytokine ,experimental Vaccine.

Introduction:
There are hetero-genus standard and standardized immune-biologics that are similar to vaccine in few or more of their features and /or their evaluation criteria exhibiting therapeutic potentials both at the levels of experimental animal models and human beings .In a previous communication it was designated as vaccine allied biologics[1].When we combine their therapeutic potentials, the designation will be" Therapeutic Vaccine Allied Biologics"[TVAB].

In the present opinion attempts were made to :
i- Review their features
ii- build up an evaluation criteria for their safety and efficacy.
iii-Propose a classification that ensemble them.

Class I :Cellular Secretions, A-Cytokines;

Cytokines are secretory hormone-like peptides or low molecular weight secretory proteins synthesized and produced by vertebrate nucleated cells like lymphocytes, macrophage ,adipocyte and epithelial cells. They are classified[2,3] into innate ,adaptive immune cytokines ,primary inflammatory, secondary inflammatory ,inflammatory and anti- inflammatory cytokines .They forms a chemical language in networking fashion for signal transduction among immune and nonimmune cells and own divers roles in immune homeostasis ,heamopoiesis ,regulation of immune and inflammatory responses Cytokines are essential biologics for medical oncology. Colony stimulating factors are of use to protect the bone marrow precursor expansion. Cytokine like type I interferon and IL2 are in common use as antitumor agents such as ;lymphomas ,multiple myeloma, renal cell carcinoma and melanoma .Unwanted co-effects are evident in case of use of IL12 as anti-tumor drug has been shown toxicity to the patients.[3].

B: Antibodies;

i-Polyclonal,

Antibodies are either of polyclonal or monoclonal nature[4].They are globular glycoprotein that found in gamma globulin area of serum electro-phoro-gram of human beings. The immunoglobulins gain their specificities to certain infectious agents ,synthesized and produced from B lymphocyte within the lymphoid organs on instu antigen stimulations. They are specific polyclonal ,since are being as net result of multiple epitope stimulations of B lymphocytes[4,5].

ii-Monoclonal:

An antigen was tempted to specific immune priming of mice using multiple dosage program in a week a part for three weeks .One week leave then the primed mice were eviscerated ,spleen saved ,macerated, and splenocyte separated .Now these splenocytes are antigen primed. myeloma lymphocyte cell line was screened for vitaly and co-cultured with these antigen primed splenocytes in cell culture with HRPTG to grow up the hybridoma cell which produce daughter cell that grown in separate cultures in which they form clones that are able to produce specific antibody homogenous physico-chemically ,genetically and immunologically such antibody is known as monoclonal antibody .Monoclonal antibody has diagnostic ,therapeutic ,and immunologic and genetic uses[6].

Antibody in Practice:

Serum technology means the techniques and assays available for making, standardizing, dispensing, releasing and marketing of immune sera. These sera are of main three classes ;immune animal sera, immune human sera and hyper-immune globulins .Disease states that needs the use of therapeutic sera are depicted in Table 1,tests for biological standardization of therapeutic sera are being detailed in Table 2.While the licensed therapeutic immune sera are tabulated in Table 3.[4,5].

Host- Immune Sera interactions;

In the immunologic sense the host-immune sera interactions means that there are epitopes within the immune sera can be as neutralization of virus, toxin or venom as well as the possible immune reactions such as the allergenic responses due to the animal derived epitopes within the immune sera which appeared as atopic or serum sickness reactions [4].

iii-Anti-cytokines;

Anti-cytokines are rather in common use for some disease conditions .Studies have shown that the anti-TNF, anti-IL6 and anti-IL5 are evident antibodies have clinical practice. However, Anti-TNF alpha have been excessively investigated both in laboratory animals and in man for bacterial, parasitic and auto-immune diseases and found to be protective Table 4.The unwanted co-effect seen is vulnerability to infection and autoimmune diseases[3].

Table 1: Disease states that may need the use of therapeutic sera.

Disease group	Therapeutic Sera
Bacterial toxin induced diseases	Diphtheria Tetanus Gas Gangrene Botulism Pertussis
Viral Diseases	Rubella Infectious hepatitis Serum hepatitis Poliomyelitis Rabies Chicken Pox Mumps Small Pox
Antibody Deficiency Syndrome	Concentrate Globulin fraction
Hematologic Diseases	Rh iso-immunization
Envenomation	Scorpion Antivenin Snake Antivenin

Table 2: The tests usable in biological standardization of therapeutic sera.

-Potencity Test
-Specificity Test
-Purity Test
-residual Toxicity
-Allergenicity Test
-Immune Protectivity Test
-Bioavailability Test
-Biohalf in-vivo test
-Determination of Shelf and Storage temperature And Stability
Determination of Best administration rout

Table 3 : The licensed therapeutic sera.

Disease	Source of Antibody	Indications
Diphtheria, Tetanus	Human, Horse	Prophylaxis, treatment
Gas Gangrene	Horse	Post exposure
Botulism	Horse	Post exposure
Snake bit	Horse	Post exposure
Scorpion sting	Horse	Post exposure
Rabies	Human	Post exposure, Vaccine
Hepatitis B	Human	Post exposure
Hepatitis A	Pooled Human Immunoglobulin	Prophylaxis, Travel
Measles	Pooled human immunoglobulin	Post exposure

From Roitt et al [4,5].

Table 4 : Anti-TNF antibodies protective in man and laboratory animals.

Bacterial Diseases
Bacterial Meningitis
Endo toxic Shock
Septic Shock
Parasitic Diseases
Cerebral Malaria
Autoimmune Diseases
Rheumatoid Arthritis
Experimental Autoimmune encephalo-meningitis

Class II receptor-anti-receptor: Immune Check Point Inhibitor:

It is a check point protein ,program death 1 PD1 recognize two legends PDL-1,and PDL-2.PDL-1 expressed on antigen presenting cells APC and many other tissues.PDL-2, expressed mainly onto APC. Engagement of PDl-1 by either legend leads to inactivation of T cells .Specific antibody to PDL-1 or its legend is effective in enhancing cancer killing T cells in mice .Several human trails have shown that PD-1 or PDL-1 blockade can limit tumor progression and reduces tumor burden in patients with advanced cancer .Such blocked can be established through the use of monoclonal antibody specific to PD-I or PDL-1or PDL-2..Check point inhibitors seek to overcome one of cancer cell main defense against the host immune system and help to keep the immune response under check. Unwanted co-effects are autoimmune disease and inflammatory reactions [7].

Class III Subunit macro-molecules :
Beta Glucans ;

Beta glucans are glucose polymers forming parts of cell wall of certain pathogenic bacteria and fungi .They are naturally occurring poly-saacharides. Beta glucans derived from different sources have shown some differences in their structures .Glucans are heterogenous group of glucose polymers consisting a back bone of B(1,6)-linked B-D-B(1,6)- with variable length and distributions.

Beta glucans exhibit an anti-infective protective influences against ;Staphylococcus aureus ,Escherichia coli ,Listeria monocytogenes ,Pneumocystis carini ,Candida albicans and Influenza virus .It is an anthrax protective in mice model .It has been tested for safety and efficacy in surgical patients at high risk for postoperative infections[8].Dose response relations for different grades of concentrations have been tested[9].

Beta glucan as a hapten has shown to be of poor immunogenicity .Conjugation with carrier protein made it immunogen and found protective against filamentous fungal pathogen in laboratory animal model. Protection seems to due to anti-glucan antibodies and never be used as a vaccine[10,11].

The features of glucan immune functions are being as ;i- activating complement system ,enhance macrophage function ,ii- augment natural killer cell functions and iii- the induction o cellular immune responses as well as iv-powerful antitumor agent[12].

Class IV: Commensal microbiome: Probiotics;

Probiotics are commensal bacteria and commensal yeasts ,that are of diverse biologic potentials .Probiotic technology covers the theme of selection of strains ,preparation of starters ,studying the strain physiology and strain immune potentials as well as cell techniques .Probiotics displayed their preventive and /or therapeutic effects through their immunogenicity, immune-adjuvant, and tumor reducing activities[13].The immune features can be through;Anti-inflammatory,antiautoimmune,anti-cancer,immunoadjuvant and vaccine delivery system[14].Upon trying to apply vaccine evaluation criteria on probiotics it showed rather similar criteria but less stringent in preparation schema[1].No reported unwanted co-effects on using probiotics.

Class V, Bacterio-therapeutics(Cancer Killing Bacteria);

Some bacterial pathogens like Streptococcus pyogenes has the anti-cancerous potentials in their natural state. Others ,however ,own such potentials after getting modification in their genetic constitutions. Two examples of genetically modified bacteria to be active as cancer killer bacteria and are being briefed[15,16] in the followings;

1-Synchronizing bacterial lysing strains that have the ability of an in-vivo delivery system that grow and release cytotoxic agents in-situe which acts as circuit engineered bacteria[15].
2-Salmonella typhimurium auxotroph AI-R that were genetically engineered to grow in viable, and necrotic tumor tissue as well as kill tumor cells in laboratory animal models [16]].Human trails are still unsuccessful.

Evaluations:

The licensed vaccine affairs for human and animals upon used as immune-prophylactants for mass vaccination programs were briefed in[17,18].Likewise ,Experimental developed vaccine for human welfare were presented in [19].What concerned with probiotics were reviewed by Shnawa [14].Cell based vaccines was reviewed in [20].Vaccine allied biologics typified by probiotics was characterized in brief through the editorial Shnawa[1].In the present opinion tempts were made to review in brief the therapeutic vaccine allied biologics focusing onto; i-Brief feature ,ii-build up oriented evaluation criteria ,Table 5,6., as well as iii- propose a classification system to them ,Table 7.

Therapeutic Vaccine Allied Biologics In Brief:

It is hetero-genus group of biologics that interplayed vaccine like potentials in both laboratory animals and man .It covers cellular secretions, subcellular, subunit macromolecules and whole cells. They , ensemble in five major classes as; Cellular secretions[cytokine ,antibodies], receptor-anti-receptor[immune check point inhibitors] ,subunit macromolecules[beta glucan], commensal microbiome[probiotics] and bacterio-therapeutics [cancer killing bacteria]. They are helpful as therapeutic agents for ;Infections ,autoimmune and neoplastic diseases .The evaluation criteria for such products subjected to that of preventive ,in addition to those that are specific to the disease.

Table 5: Evaluation Parameters for preventive Vaccines

Evaluation Criteria[17]	Viral[22]	Bacterial[21]	Fungal[23,24]	Neoplastic[25]
Understanding disease	U	U	U	U
Understanding disease cause	U	U	U	[U]
Preparation of vaccine candidate	P	P	P	P
Laboratory Animal				
Safety	+	+	+	+
Antigenicity	+	+	+	+
Immunogenicity	+	+	+	+
Phase I S	+	+	+ 2V	+ 1V
Phase II S A	+	+	-	+ 1V
Phase III S A PT	+	+	-	+ 1V

U = Understandable   [U] = Questionable understanding
P = Prepared
S+Safety   A = Antigenicity   PT = Protectivity   V = Vaccine

Table 6 : Evaluation Criteria For Therapeutic Vaccine Allied Biologics.

Bacterial[21]	Viral [22]	Fungal [23,24]	Neoplastic [25]	Conclusion
1-Reduction of bacterial load 2-Immune conversion 3-Recovery duration 4-Recurrent Episode	1-reduction of Viral load 2-Immune conversion 3-Efficacy	NDY	1-Reduction of lesion size 2-Durable stable disease 3-Response in total tumor burden 4-Response in presence of new lesion	Bacterial and viral reach clinical trail Fungal not defined yet[NDY] Neoplastic reach in these examples but ,they reach clinical in others.

NDY=not yet defined

Table 7 : Classes of Vaccine Allied Biologics.

Classes	Representative

Cellular secretions	A-Cytokines
	B-Antibodies
	  i-Polyclonal
	  ii-Monoclonal
	  iii-Anti-cytokines

Receptor –Anti-receptor	Immune check point inhibitors
Subunit macromolecules	Beta glucan
Commensal microbiome	Probiotics
Bacterio-therapeutics	Cancer killing bacteria

References
1-Shnawa IMS,2016,Vaccine allied biologics, IJVV ,2(2):00024.
2-Shnawa IMS,2016,Oral Epithelial cytokines,IJVV,2(2):00026.
3-Mantovani A, Dinarello CA , Ghezzi P,2000,Pharmacology of Cytokines,Oxford university Press,Oxford,233-237.
4-Roitt I,Brostoff J ,Male D,2001,Immunology 6th ed.Mosby,London,285.
5-Banker DD,1982,Modern Practice In Immunization ,Popula Praskashan,Bombay,40-70.
6-Abraham E, Wudrink R , Silverman H et al., 1995,Efficacy and safety of monoclonal antibodies to TNF alpha with systemic syndrome.A randomized double blind ,multicenter clinical trials ,JAAMA,273;934-941.
7-Abbas AK ,Lichtman NH ,Pillai ,2013,Cellular And Molecular Immunology ,Elseveirs Saunders,Philadelphia,321,391.
8-Bromuro ,Torosantucci P ,Chainict P,Conti S,Polonelli L Casson A ,2002,Interplay between protective and inhibitory antibody dictates the outcomes of experimentally disseminated candidiasis in relation to Candida albicans vaccine,Inf.Immun.,70:5462-5470.
9-Torosatucci A ,Bornuro C, Chiani P ,De F,Berti F,Galli C ,Norelli F,Bellucci C,2005,A Novel glycol-conjugate vaccine against fungal pathogens,J.Exp.Med.,202:597-606.
10-Babineau TJ,Marceas P,Swails W,Kenler A,Bistian B,frose RF,1994,randomized PhaseI/II trials of macrophage PGG glucan in high risk surgical patients.,Arch.Surg.,230:601-609.

11-Babinaeu TJ,hackfor A ,kenler A,Bristian B ,Frose RA faircheld PG et al.1994,A phase I multicenter randomized plcebo controlled study of three dosage of PGGglucan in high risk surgical patients,Arch.Surg.,129:1204-1210.

12Akramanone D,Kondrotas A,Didziapetriene J,Kerelaitis E,2007,Effect of Beta glucan on the immune system,Medicinia (Kaunas),43(8):597-606.

13-Reid G,1999,Scientific bases for probiotic strains of lactobacilli. ,Appl.Env .Microbiol .65(9):3763-3766.

14-Shnawa IMS,2016,The Immune Potentials of Probiotics,Int.J.Vacc.Imm.Sys.,1(1):14-18.

15-Omar Din M ,Danino,T,,Prindle A ,Skalak M ,Selimkhanov J,Allen E,Atolia E,Bhatia SN,Hasty J,2016,Synchronized cycles of bacterial lysis in-vivo delivery,Nature 636:81-85.

16-Uchuonova A , Zhao M , zhang Y,Weinigel M,Kong K ,Hoffman RM ,2012,Cancer killing Salmonella imaged by multiphoton Tomography in live mice,Anticancer. Res.32:4331-4338.

17-NIH,1998,Understanding Vaccines,NIH,Publication No.98-4219,23.

18-Shnawa IMS,2016,Vaccinology At A Glance,Lap lambert academic Publications,

19-Shnawa IMS 2016,Vaccinology Letters :A Treatise Concerning The Experimental Vaccine ,IITE,USA.

20- Shnawa IMS,2017,Dendritic Cell based Vaccine for human tuberculosis,IJVI,2(1):1-6.

21-Lorenzo-Gomez MF ,Padilla-fernandez B,Garcia-Cardin FJ,Miron-Canella JA,Gii-Viceenle A ,Nito-Huerotes A ,Silva-Abuin JM,2013.Evaluation of therapeutic vaccines for prevention of recurrent urinary tract infections versus prophylactic treatment with antibiotics,Int..Urogynecol.J.,24:127-134.

22-Spaans JN,Routy J-P,Trembaly C, et al.,2012,Optimizing the efficiency of therapeutic for HIV vaccine trial :A case for CTN 123,Trials In Vaccinology,1:21-26.

23-riva A,Hohl TM,2015,Calnexin Bridges the gap toward a pan-fungal vaccine,Cell-Host and Microbes,17:421-423.

24-Nanjappa SG,Kelin BS,23014,Vaccine –immunity against fungal infection ,Curr.opin .Immunol.,28:27-33.

25-Wolchok JD,Hoos A,ODay S, et al.,2009,guidelines for the evaluation of immunotherapy activity in solid tumors,Immune related response,Criteria,Clin.Canc.Res.,15(@#):7412-7419.

VACCINE ALLIED BIOLOGICS -II
One of the themes that are longly born in mind ,those concerning " Vaccine versus Probiotics" .Then, if it is feasible to raise a question such as" Could we consider Probiotic as a vaccine ,since they have an in-common indications ,applications and/or attributes ,Table 1.The common affairs are rather more than the different affairs. Thus ,I think that they are forms of bio- therapeutics owning vaccine like potentials or one can say that they are vaccine-allied biologics.

Table 1 : Characteristics of vaccine versus probiotics

Features	Probiotics	Vaccines
Starter	Certain commensal bacteria	Pathogens or their subunits
Specificity	Nonspecific in most cases	Specific in most cases
Evaluation attitude	Less stringent for human favor	Stringent for human favor
Dispensing	Drug-like dispensing menu	Needs special dispensing menu
Indication	Biotherapy of various immune defects in man and animals	Immunoprphylaction
Use	On individual basis more than massive	Massive use rather than individual cases
Disease nature	Infectious and non-infectious	Infectious ,epidemic and pandemic threat or on travel to epidemic or endemic areas
Mode of action	Bacteriocin ,immunomodulatory ,anticancerous	Based on affinity of B and T memory cells
Side Effect	No appearent side effect	Mild short duration like fever and ill
Failure	Due to probiotic or host born causes	Due to vaccine or host born causes

References

1-Banker D D,1980,Modren Practice In Immunization ,Popular Prakshan ,Bomby ,India.

2-Kaufmann,SHE,2004,Novel Vaccination Strategies,Wiley-VCH,Germany.

3- Kumar H,Salminen S , Vergagen H, Rowland I , Heimbach,J , Banares S ,Young T , Nomoto K,Lalonde M,2015,Probiotics and prebiotics road to market,Curr.Opin.Biotech.,32:99-103.

4-Quigley EMM,2016,Leaky gut-Concept or clinical entity,Curr.Opin.Gastroenterol.,22:74-79.

THE IMMUNE POTENTIALS OF PROBIOTICS
ABSTRACT

Probiotics are vaccine allied biologics, vaccine adjuvants ,oral vaccines ,vaccine prim-boost and, vaccine delivery systems .They are formed from commensal bacteria and commensal yeasts .Such candidate preparation are developed and evaluated in a way similar to that of vaccine development and evaluations with less stringent control measures . They can be of therapeutic and preventive uses both for infectious and lympho-proliferative diseases.

INTRODUCTION

The concept of using bacteria for treatment and prevention as well as health insurance is not modern but it is rooted back to 1930s of the 20th century . However in the current days there is a renewal of the interest of probiotic use.Probiotic technology covers the theme of selection of strains, preparation of starters ,studying the strain physiology and strain immune potentials well as cell immobilization techniques .Probiotics displayed their preventive and /or therapeutic influences through their immunogenicity, immune-modulating as well as tumor reducing activities[1].The objective of the present mini-review was to introduce probiotics as an immune-prophylactants and immunotherapeutics

CONCEPT

Originally ,probiotics as a term is referred to a secretory product of a microbe that promotes the growth of the other microbe living within the same ecologic niche Such term means in the straight English language" For the life"[2].Parker in 1975[3] have demonstrate that probioics denoted to substances of microbe that posses positive role in restoration of the equilibrium of the intestinal microflora.Fuller in 1989[4],have been assured that probiotics means microbes which have certain biological and immunological determinants by which they can pass through mouth till intestines (ceccum).

FEATURES

The immune-biologic features of the probiotic microbes are being depicted in Table 1.They adhere to the intestinal and uro-genital cells and reduce pathogens through steric- hindrance ,production of bio-surfactants ,production of biocines and competition for nutrients .After instillation in the intestines and vagina they persist for three days in the intestines and seven weeks in the vagina .Some probiotic strains resist the micro-bicides and spermicide activities in intestines and vagina respectively.They formed coaggregates,biofilms and overgrow other pathogens,though they are nonpathogens.Probiotic bacteria are mainly from Lactobacilli and bifidobacter, while probiotic yeasts are from the genera Saccharomyces and Candida.[1,4].

Table 1: Characteristic features of the probiotics[1,4].

Nature	Description
Physiologic	-Acid tolerance - Digestive juce tolerance -Antibody tolerance -Bile acid resistance -Production of volatile acid to restore the equilibrium of microflora -Resist killing by blood -Compets for nutrients - Host compatibility -Persist and overgrow other microbes
Immunologic	-Adhere to mucous membrane -Form biofilm -Reduce pathogens -Reduce cancer growth -Induce immune response events -Acts as an immune modulant

MODE OF ACTION[5,6,7]

Probiotics performed their immune-biologic functions via several immune mechanisms like;
i-Adherence and colonization of mucosal surfaces.
Ii-Competition for nutrients.
iii-Antagonism
iv-Production of Organic acids
v-Co-aggregation and overgrowth
vi-Immune mechanisms like antibody responses induction of cytokine network ,immune-adjuvant action ,tumor reducing ability.

TECHNOLOGY[8,9,10]:

Cell immobilization techniques have pre-requests, such pre-requests are being stated in the following;

i-Candidate Probiotics ;After the starter of the probiotic microbes are being propagated and thoroughly evaluated using a series of evaluation parameters then they are ready for loading to a specified carrier.

ii-The chemical nature of the carrier materials are heterogeneous including, polysaachardes ,starch ,dextran and agarose derivatives .Alternatively ,proteins can be of use as loading carriers such as gelatin , albumin and resins.

iii-Cell immobilization; Cell immobilization processes are, loading, linking , entrapping of microbial probiotic cells and encapsulation.

iv-Entrapping; Probiotic cells are trapped inside synthetic tissues made from gel such as polycrylamide ,K-carrageenan and calcium alginate. Though ,calcium alginate ,carrrageenan and starch are preferred.

v-Encapsulation System; The use of starch as an encapsulation system for probiotics will be as in the following steps;

i-Large granules are treated with enzyme to obtain porous structure.

ii-If starch found as amylose it should be solubilized and cooled .

iii-The treated starch is of use as carrier in which probiotic suspension derived from broth culture media is precipitated on the surface of the starch granules to fill up the porous structures allowing chemical and physical bounding to starch surface

iv-The final product is lyophilized to be obtained in dried form.

CAPSULE MIGRATION[8.9,10]:

The capsule production in this way is known as simple precipitation and it is most sound in use and of high efficiency for production of coats for this stable and resistant capsules. The probiotic starch encapsulation is resistant to action of acids ,juces and enzymes on passage through; mouth, esophagous ,stomach and small intestines ,when the capsule reach colon it hydrolyzed and probiotic materials are released after grow and increase in numbers due starch formation by the colonic bacteria and by the probiotic growing cells.

EVALUATION CRITERIA

Both of the small and large scale production of probiotics should fulfills several evaluation criteria[8,9,10] which includes the followings
i-Reliability ,strain nature.
ii-Viability'.
iii-Adhesion Ability.
iv-Antagonistic Activity.
v-Safety., proof to be non-toxic
vi-Stability. ,genetic back ground.
vii-Immunogenicity, antibody and cytokine response.
viii-Immuno-modulating activity.
ix- Immune Protectivity.
x-Tumor Regression Ability.

PROBIOTIC HOST IMMUNE RESPONSES[11,12]:

When the probiotic cell clones reached , thereby in the colon they are taken up by M cells onto the surface lining of the Pyres patches or across the normal epithelium overlying the lamina properia .In pyres patches the M cells transport the intact probiotic cells to the phagocytes to be phagocytized by the antigen presenting cells(APC) the macrophage and dendritic cells. The APC process and express the antigenic peptide along with MHCII molecules onto its surface. The peptide MHC combinations on the surface of APC ,in turn presented to T cells through helper effect will activate B lymphocyte to grow ,proliferate, expand and then differentiated to plasma cells. While if the probiotic antigen crosses the normal epithelium ,it will has the potential to activate the lamina properia T cells and induce T cell immune responses.

When the mucosal immune responses are stimulated ,primed T and B lymphocytes migrate through lymphatic vessels ,then entered the peripheral blood circulation via the thoracic lymph duct. Extravasation do happened to the immune cells and then enrolled in traffic ,migrate and homed into the common mucosal immune system compartments ;lamina properia ,respiratory tissue ,uro-genital tissue ,mammary and salivary glands .Such migration is referred to as an IgA cycle. Though on the contrary to the migration and homing stories . If the probiotic cells are bounded to epithelial cells, then they will have only local effects on the gut.

They are unable to induce IgA cycle or to increase CD4+ T cells. Their effects only exerted through the induction of cytokine release by the stimulated cells without the need for antigen processing. Probiotics, during the passage through the gut ,they will raise up S IgA, cytokine responses as well as they will induce their own specific mucosal antibody responses of the gut .

PROBIOTICS VERSUS VACCINE :

Probiotics are vaccine and vaccine allied Biologics. There are some similarities and difference in between them[13].

Table 2 gives rather logical comparison between probiotic and vaccines;

Features	Probiotics	Vaccines
Starter	Certain commensal bacteria	Pathogens or their subunits
Specificity	Nonspecific in most cases	Specific in most cases
Evaluation attitude	Less stringent for human favor	Stringent for human favor
Dispensing	Drug-like dispensing menu	Needs special dispensing menu
Indication	Biotherapy of various immune defects in man and animals	Immunoprphylaction
Use	On individual basis more than massive	Massive use rather than individual cases
Disease nature	Infectious and non-infectious	Infectious ,epidemic and pandemic threat or on travel to epidemic or endemic areas
Mode of action	Bacteriocin,immunomodulatory ,anticancerous	Based on affinity of B and T memory cells
Side Effect	No appearent side effect	Mild short duration like fever and ill
Failure	Due to probiotic or host born causes	Due to vaccine or host born causes

BIOTHERAPY[14,15,16,17,18,19,] :

Probiotics have been tempted in rather many therapeutic protocols of human and animal diseases to modulate immunity in autoimmune diseases like rheumatoid arthritis, inflammatory bowel disease and, allergic diseases like atopic dermatitis .They, also posses the potential of tumor growth reduction and prevention of diarrhea and urinary tract infection. Diarrhea occur in around 20% of patients whom received antibiotic treatment. Antibiotic associated diarrhea results from microbial imbalance that lead to decrease in the endogenous micro-flora that is usually responsible for colonization resistance and decrease in colonic capacity for fermentation. It has been found that probiotic treatment restore patient normal state in a range of 5 to 17%. Several controlled randomized trails have shown the beneficial effects of probiotics in therapeutic and preventive measures of gastroenteritis patients. In a group of 116 patients with IBD were given probiotic preparations .It was found that it is effective as that of Mesasalalin (R) in inducing remission and preventing relapse of IBD patients .

IMMUNE POTENTIALS[20,21,22]

Probiotics are responsible for about 70% of human immune responses and anti-cancerous ability[18].They have anti-inflammatory influences[19] .Probiotics posses vaccine adjuvant effects and vaccine prime-boost potentials as well as vaccine and vaccine delivery system as well ,Tables 3 and 4.

Table 3:Probiotic vaccine adjuvants.

Immune potentials	References
Normal mucosal adjuvant,	22
Probiotic Lactobacillus adjvant	23
T cell immunomodulatory	24

Table 4: Probiotic vaccine.

Immune Potentials	Reference
Probiotic oral vaccine	25
Probiotic oral live vaccine and vaccine delivery system	26
Probiotic based malaria vaccine	27
Drinkable HIV vaccine	28
Specific probiotic boost antibody response to oral and systemic vaccine	29

CONCLUDING REMARKS :

Finally to put-forward a concluding remarks to this mini-review one may state the basic immune features of probiotics as in the following;
i-Anti-inflammatory.
ii-Anti-autoimmune disease.
iii-Anti-cancerous.
iv-Immuonogen.
v-Immuno- adjuvant.
vi-Vaccine.
vii-The boost part of the prime boost protocol.
viii-Vaccine delivery System.

REFERENCES :

1-Reid G,1999,Scientific bases for probiotic strains of Lactobcillus ,Appl .Env. Microbiol,65 (9):3763-3766.
2 – Lilly DM,Stillwell RJ,1965,Probiotic growth promoting factors produced by microorganisms,Science,147;747-748.
3-Parker DS ,1975,Probiotics the other half of the Antibiotic story,Anim.Nutr.health,29;4-8.
4-Fuller R, 1989,Probiotics In Man And Animals,J.Appl.Bacteriol.,70:443-459.
5-AlderberthI, Ahren S,1996,Aannose specific adherence mechanism in Lactobacillus plantarum conferring binding to human colonic cell line HT29,Appl.Env. MIcrobiol,,62:2244-2251.
6-Arunachalam,K ,Gill HS,2000,Enhancement of natural immune function by dietary consumpti byBifidobacterium lactis (HN019) Eur.J.Cli. Nutr,54(4):187190.
7-Barefoot,SF,Kaenhammer TR 1984,Purification and characterization of Lactobacillus acidophilus bacteriocinB Atimicrob.Agents. Chemother.,26(3):328-324.
8-Chiabata I,Tosa T ,Sato T,1986,Methods for Cell immobilization,In Dermain AL,Solomon NA eds, Manual of Industrial Microbiology And Biotechnology.American Society of Micrbiology,Washington D.C.
9-Cassidy MB,Lee ,Trevors JT,1996,Environmental Application of Immobilized cell2, J.Ind.Microbiol.,16,79-101.
10-Tanaka A, Nakajima H,1990,Application of immobilized growing cells ,Adv.Biochem.Eng.Biotechnol.42,;97-131.
11-Perdigon G,Vintini E,Alvarez S,Medina M, Mededici M,1999,Study of the possible mechanisms involoved in mucosal immune system activation by lactic acid bacteria,J .Dair.Sci.,82:1108-1114.

12-Perdigon G ,Alvarez S,Rachid M,Aguero G,Gobbato N,1995,Immune system stimulation by probiotics.J.Dair.Sci.78:1597-1606.
13- Shnawa,IMS,2016,Vaccine allied biologics ,IVVO,2(2) :00024 .
14-Martueau PR, de Verse M, Cellier CJ ,Schrezenmeir J,2001,Protection from gastro-intestinal diseases with the use of probiotics ,Am.J.Nut.73(Suppl):4305 4365.
15-World Gastroenterology Organization Handbook on Gut Microbe,2014
16-Allen S analysis of 63 studies show that probiotics are safe J ,Martinez EG, Gregio GV,Dems LF,2010,A metanalysis of 63 studies show that probiotics are safe and have clear benefit in treatment of infectious diarrhea ,when used with rehydration therapy,Cochrane Data base system Rev.,Epub. No,10.
17Hayes SR,Vargas AJ,2016,Probiotics for prevention of pediatric Antibiotic associated diarrhea,Explore (NY),Aug 27 2016,PMID:27688016.
18-Baroja ML,Kirjavainen PV,Hekmat S,Reid G,2007,Anti-Infammatory effect of yogurt in inflammatory bowel disease patients,Clin.Exp.Immnunol.149(3):470-279.
19-Probiotic Org.,2015,21 Amazing facts about Probiotics.
20-Kopp-HoolihanIssue,L,2001,Prophylactic And TherapeuticUses of Probiotics:A Review,J.Am. Dietettic. Ass.,1:1-15.
21-Meydani S, Ha W,2000,Immunological Effects of yoghourt,Am.J.Clin.Nutr.71;861-872.
22-Licciardi PV,Tang ML,2011,Vaccine adjuvant properties of probiotic bacteria ,Discov.Med. 12(67);525-533.

23-Inc-Kanada A ,Stojanoric M ,Marinokovic E ,Becker E ,Dojokic R, Schuerer N, Hegemann JH,Barisani-Asenbauer T, 2016, A probiotic adjuvant Lactobacillus rhamosus enhances specific immune responses after ocular mucosal immunization with Chlamydial polymorphic membrane protein C,Plose One Sep,16 2016 dio,org/10 1371.

24-Chattha KS,Viasova AN,Kandasamy S ,Rajashekara G,saif LJ ,2013,divergent immunomodulating effects of probiotics on T cell responses to oral Human rotavirus infection in neonatal Gnotobiotic piglet Disease Model ,J.Immunol. ,191:2446-2456.

25-Tetro J,2016,Probiotic may be the new vaccines,A Blog,Huffpost living canal,Dec.11,2016.

26-Boersms WJA,Shaw M ,Claassen E,2000,probiotic bacteria as live oral vaccine Lactobacillus as the versatile Delivery vechile, In Fuller R ,Predigon G (eds), Probiotis 3 ,walter Kluwer Academic Publisher,234-270.

27-Ngwa CJ, Praddel G ,2015,Coming Soon ,Probiotic based malarial vaccine ,trends ,Parasitol.,31(1);2-4.

28-Naguyen T,2014,Research has radical idea for drinkable probiotic HIV vaccine ,Washington Post.

29-McDonald TT,Bell I,2010,Probiotics and the immune response to vaccines. Proc.Nat.Soc.,69(3):442-446.

SOURCE REFERENCE

Chapter One:
1- Shnawa,IMS,2014,Introductory Overview Vaccinology Course/Biotechnology students. College of Biotechnology ,Qasim University.

Chapter Two
2- Shnawa IMS,2017,Bacterin InducedPathogenic Lapin And Murine Cryoglobulin,Current Trends in Vaccines And Vaccinology,1(1)

Chapter Three:
3- Shnawa I M S,2014,Individual Variations And Human Herd Immunity,J.Nat.Sci.Res.4 (8):31-38.

Chapter Four:
4- Shnawa I M S,2017,Dendritic Cell Based Vaccine For Human Tuberculosis.Int.J.Vacc.Immun.Syst.2(1):1-6.

Chapter Five:
5- Shnawa I M S,2017,Vaccine Allied Biologics,Int.J.Vacc.Immu.Syst.2(2):13-19.

Chapter Six:
6- Shnawa I M S 2016,Editorial,Vaccine Allied Biologics,Int.J Vacc.Vaccination 2(2):00024.

Chapter Seven:
7- Shnawa I M S ,2016,Immune Potentials of Probiotics,Int.J.Vacc.Immun.Syst. 1(1):14-18.

www.ingramcontent.com/pod-product-compliance
Lightning Source LLC
Chambersburg PA
CBHW070410230526
45471CB00006B/2742